C^{The}hange'll
Do You Good

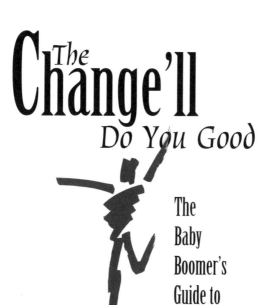

The
Baby
Boomer's
Guide to
Menopause

Dr. Carol Schulen

Carol Schulen

DCS
Publishing
Chicago, Illinois

Published by DCS PUBLISHING
33 West Huron, Suite 809
Chicago, IL 60610

Publisher's Cataloging-in-Publication Data
Schulen, Carol.
    The change'll do you good : the baby boomer's guide to menopause /
    Carol Schulen -- Chicago, IL : DCS Publishing., 2000.
        p.   cm.
    ISBN 0-9672352-0-0

    1. Menopause–popular works. I. Title.   II. Baby boomer's guide to
    menopause.   III. Change will do you good.
RG186 .S38   2000   99-62714
612.665   dc—21   CIP

PROJECT COORDINATION BY JENKINS GROUP, INC.

02 01 00 99 ᴜ⃰ 5 4 3 2 1

Printed in the United States of America

To Vance
my husband and best friend,
and
to our children,
Nancy, Lori, Tracey, and Dina

CONTENTS

CHECKLISTS

1.

AND NOW FOR SOMETHING COMPLETELY DIFFERENT

This time, like all times, is a very good one,
if we but know what to do with it.
—RALPH WALDO EMERSON

❧

THE BABY BOOM GENERATION! We have watched the progress of this important segment of our population with great interest as they have reached each milestone: preschool, elementary school, puberty, high school, college, the work force. Each step has been marked with the characteristics of this unique group. They are independent, unwilling to accept the wisdom of the past, and prepared to forge new paths to create history on their own terms. They openly discuss more, communicate more, and argue more. Now a new milestone is on the horizon. Middle age! And for half of the "boomers," the women, that means menopause with all of the myths that surround it. Already this once taboo subject has become the object of public discussion. And if the past is any indication, some of the old myths and beliefs will fall.

In 1991 with the release of Gail Sheehy's book, *The Silent Passage,* the communication floodgates began to open and the topic of menopause moved into the mainstream of everyday conversation. With her powerful and moving description, "a lonely and emotionally draining experience. . . virtually nothing prepares most women for this mysterious and momentous transition," she set the stage for a more candid and honest discussion. For many women this helped crystalize their views.

It also brought to the forefront of consciousness and communication the prevailing opinion of the day in a way that allowed it to be examined and challenged. In other words, no longer is the passage silent.

Not only that, something else became quite evident. Menopause was defined almost exclusively by symptoms with a medical focus, a one-dimensional view that pathologizes women's natural aging process. The not surprising consequence of this very limited view was that menopause was thought of as a medical disorder, an inevitable, chronic disease cured by hormone replacement. Further, following that line of reasoning, every woman over fifty years of age became a patient. Authors, medical or otherwise, who have addressed the subject have depicted menopause as a chronic disease and then described it as an illness with no real regard for the presence or absence of distressful symptoms. This natural life process has been forced into a "disease model" and that means it can or should be "cured."

Perhaps one reason this model has appealed to so many is that it allowed emotional problems to be attributed to a hormonal deficiency which is, of course, a medical problem, rather than seeing it as psychological one. To many people, medical problems are more acceptable than psychological problems. While there may be some general misunderstandings of psychology, the attraction of this model has its basis in our culture. Physical symptoms of a disease are more easily treated with prescription medicine and therefore offer a passive solution. Psychological problems, on the other hand, often carry a stigma and are more difficult to treat. Psychological problems are more difficult to treat because treatment almost always requires an active participative role by the patient.

Researchers have recently been able to establish the fact that specific psychological treatment, such as thought and behavior change, do have direct and lasting effect on physical symptoms. Above all, this approach yields virtually no detrimental side affects. However, it is much "easier" to take a pill than it is to change behavior or lifestyle and American culture in particular gravitates toward the instant gratification afforded by the medical model.

Relating the medical model to menopause implies that menopause is a disease that requires medical treatment. In addition, focusing on medical treatment tends to divert attention from the other, lifestyle-related options that have proven equally valuable for preventing or managing the symptoms. For most Americans, taking a pill is much easier than undertaking those behavior changes, like smoking cessation, nutritional management, consistent exercise, etc., that would be required.

This is beginning to change. The baby boom generation, known for breaking new trails, making its own way, is defying the past. It is not accepting menopause as a disease. And with good reason. For in the year 2046 a larger percentage than ever before will reach their 100th birthday. Is it any wonder that they show concern for their future health? With the information we have, and based on the technology available today, the baby boom generation will not only live longer than any other generation in history, they will also be the first to have the ability to establish influence over their aging process. They will live longer, they know it, and therefore they can and will plan for it. Their quality of life in later years will depend largely upon the actions they take now. In other words, adopting health behaviors.

2.

HEALTH BEHAVIORS

To be or not to be . . .
—WILLIAM SHAKESPEARE

࿇

HEALTH BEHAVIORS CAN BEST BE DEFINED as the things you do to remain healthy. These are things such as regular exercise and attention to nutrition. Any behavior that increases the likelihood of good health can be considered a health behavior. One of my former clients, Joan (56), put it this way: "There was a time when I couldn't envision myself restrained in a car by a seat belt. And now I can't imagine it any other way!" The little things you do each day to keep yourself healthy add up over time. Simple things like using seat belts while driving or riding in a car, getting enough rest, and reducing stress are health behaviors. For women, health behaviors become even more important as they approach menopause. The change that women experience between the ages of 45 and 55 is not merely a change from reproductive to nonreproductive any more than the onset of menstruation was merely a change from nonreproductive to reproductive. Both are a collection of changes. The parallel developmental phases of beginning menstruation and the end of it occur naturally in the life of every woman who lives long enough. However, prior to menopause, nature provides its primary childcare givers with good health. Therefore, many women have been able to take good health for granted. For instance, Janet (51) said:

> When I was in my twenties, I never gave my health a second thought. I had endless energy. With three children under the age of five, I really didn't have time to think about my health. Now, my youngest in college, I'm willing to begin taking care of myself.

Menopause, a kind of wake-up call, marks the time when women must increase health behaviors in order to maintain their good health.

Now that you have a sense of what health behavior is and why it is more important now than it has been in the past, the question is what to do about it. As always, the toughest task is just to get started. Participating in new health behaviors requires a new way of thinking; an active reduction in irrational thoughts. Ask yourself, "Is it rational to think that you can lead a sedentary life of poor nutrition for eighty to one hundred years and remain highly functional?" The answer is obviously no. Any other conclusion is irrational. In order to have a positive influence on your aging process, the first step is to recognize and change irrational thought patterns that lead to irrational behavior. So let's get started. *The Change'll Do You Good.*

3.

MENOPAUSE: WHAT'S IT ALL ABOUT?

Deep into that darkness peering,
long I stood there wondering, fearing . . .
—EDGAR ALLAN POE

⚘

T HE WORD "MENOPAUSE" REFERS to the end of menstrual bleeding. This can occur for some women as early as their late thirties and early forties while for others there will be no change until their mid-fifties. The average age when menstruation ceases is 50.5 years. For Cindy (51), "It began with night sweats, after several months my periods became irregular. That lasted for a couple of years before my periods stopped all together. Now I'm back to night sweats."

Diane (51) recalled:

> I could feel myself get so warm I thought I was going to burn up! My face would flush and then I would become soaking wet. It happened several times a day. At first I didn't want to admit to myself that it was menopause. I tried denial but it didn't work.

You will, of course, experience menopause in your own way just as you experienced your menstrual cycle in your own way. As you think about changes in your normal cycle, you may wonder what normal is. It is what has been normal for you usually up to your mid to late forties. Menopausal changes do not just happen all at once!

The term that describes the time when these changes are occurring is peri-menopause. It is at this time that hormonal levels have gradually decreased to the point that your menstrual cycle becomes irregular; varying noticeably from what has been normal for you. Your periods may fluctuate in length and intensity; they can be short, long, heavy, light or any combination. You will find you can no longer predict with any accuracy when you will have your period, how heavy it will be, or how long it will last. If this is of concern, take comfort in the fact that the peri-menopausal phase usually lasts two to three years. The phase to which you are moving is the "post-menopausal" phase. The term "post menopausal" refers to women who have not had a period for twelve months or more.

The transition from reproductive to nonreproductive does not occur overnight. It actually begins two to four years before you recognize any irregularity and continues for years after. The ovaries begin to slow down as they begin to produce less estrogen. Eventually the production of estrogen becomes so low that periods cease entirely. Some find the transition to be easy and uneventful; others suffer troublesome symptoms such as hot flashes, night sweats and vaginal dryness. As many as 80 percent of women experience some degree of the symptoms described, with only five to fifteen percent experiencing symptoms severe enough to require professional attention. For most, the mild symptoms will be accepted as part of the natural transition, just as the onset of menstruation was accepted with little or no medical intervention. Both are an integral part of the natural cycle of life.

4.

MENOPAUSE, I PRESUME

*How much pain have cost us
the evils which have never happened.*
—THOMAS JEFFERSON

～

FOR MOST WOMEN THE FIRST SIGNS of menopause appear between the ages of forty-five and fifty. Some, however, begin to experience symptoms as early as their late thirties and others as late as their mid-fifties. Menopause is a gradual process signaled by a change in your menstrual cycle. If your cycle has never been regular, those first signs may be more difficult to detect. This period of time, peri-menopause, commences as hormone levels decrease. From this point on, your cycle will noticeably change until menstruation completely ceases. The symptoms during peri-menopause mimic symptoms commonly associated with your regular menstrual cycle, but they differ in both length and intensity. If you experienced mild or minimal symptoms during your regular menstrual cycle, you will likely experience mild or minimal menopausal symptoms. On the other hand, if you have suffered severe symptoms during menstruation, you are more likely to experience symptoms of greater intensity during menopause. One word of caution. Often people confuse symptoms of menopause with symptoms more properly associated with poor health or the results arising from other life events. Samantha (47) complained, "I seem to forget things more often, things I'm sure I wouldn't have forgotten ten years ago!" At the time, Samantha was getting her oldest daughter off to her first year of college, it's no wonder she was preoccupied! Keep in mind that menopause is only one aspect of your life. If, for example, you find you are depressed look at other events that have occurred in your life. If you have a history of depression prior to menopause, you are likely to be depressed during menopause as well. That does not make depression a symptom of menopause. In fact, the symptoms of menopause can be clearly defined.

Symptoms that distinguish menopause from the regular menstrual cycle:

hot flashes
night sweats
vaginal dryness/atrophy

Symptoms often associated with but not related to menopause:

anxiety	anger
depression	increased stress
insomnia	irritability
nervousness	mood swings
fatigue	hopelessness
low self-esteem	lower sex drive

Jean (50) had a terrible time! Her symptoms were difficult to describe. To her it seemed that no one understood her situation. At times she felt anxious and at other times she felt nervous and depressed. Upon further analysis, she learned that these were the same symptoms she had experienced during her menstrual cycle, only now the symptoms were more erratic. Remember, if you encountered some of these "associated but not related" symptoms during your menstrual cycle, you can still expect to experience those same symptoms during menopause. You will find, however, that the duration and intensity will vary.

5.

HOT FLASHES

Some say the world will end in fire,
Some say in ice.
From what I've tasted of desire
I hold with those who favor fire.
—ROBERT FROST

A HOT FLASH, ONE OF THE SYMPTOMS that women most often complain about during menopause, is an episode that ranges from feeling very warm to a feeling of intense heat. It causes no damage, only discomfort. These episodes come on unexpectedly and vary in degree. Sometimes one needs only to remove a sweater or jacket to gain relief; other times one breaks into a profuse sweat and the level of discomfort is much greater. Although we know little about the causes of hot flashes, there is evidence that coffee, alcohol, and cigarette smoking trigger hot flashes and increase their severity. The frequency and intensity of hot flashes vary widely. Most last for 2 to 3 minutes. Hot flashes that occur during the night are often referred to as night sweats. Night sweats vary in frequency and duration as well. Some women sleep right through them, others wake up soaking from perspiration.

During my research I found that women experienced hot flashes in different ways. For some hot flashes present a minor irritation. For example, Karen (50) related her experience:

> At first it really bothered me. I kept waking up and I didn't know what to do. After a while I became used to it. During the night, when I begin to feel a wave of heat, I throw the covers off. After a few minutes I feel cold and pull the covers back. It happens several times during the night. Now I carry out the routine without fully waking up. Within a few minutes I'm back under the cover and sleeping again.

Some women have a different view. When asked about her menopausal experience, Cindy (53) replied. "It sucks!"

"What about it bothers you most?" I inquired.

She responded:

> Hot flashes. It really bothers me at night. I can't get any sleep! I feel tired during the day because I keep waking up all night. Waking up is bad enough, but I'm soaking wet! During the day I find it annoying but I can deal with that. But at night it's just too much!

The difference in Karen and Cindy's experience was the way they felt about it. What worked for Karen would not work for Cindy. For Karen, further evaluation showed that lifestyle (i.e., caffeine reduction) and adaptive behavior changes (i.e., reduce temperature, clothing, etc.) would reduce the number and intensity of hot flashes. Cindy found that sleeping became less turbulent once she changed her perspective from "Look what's happening to me!" to "What can I do to alleviate the symptoms?"

If you find you experience hot flashes or night sweats, explore your options. You may wish to seek the help of a professional psychologist. A psychologist can evaluate your lifestyle and recommend behavior changes. In addition to helping you to bring about difficult behavior changes such as eliminating caffeine, alcohol, and nicotine, a professional can also help with perspective changes as well. Such behavior and perspective changes, though difficult, will alleviate distress during menopause. Yes, that means if you want to reduce hot flashes in both number and intensity, you'll have to switch to decaf and quit smoking. Very difficult changes that may require professional help.

Help from a professional psychologist is but one of your options. You may wish to see your physician who will probably prescribe estrogen to relieve hot flashes (see Chapter 34). Or, check out J.A. Duke's *The Green Pharmacy*. Duke suggests easing menopausal symptoms with alternatives such as foods, herbal supplements, and phytoestrogens (from plants). Many women have found relief from these remedies. A word of caution: when you choose these alternatives, you choose a path of uncharted terrain since at this time these products are neither standardized nor regulated. Thus you can not be sure that the dosage is as stated on the label or that the product is consistent from one package to another. In addition, over-the-counter self-help products are recommended for moderate symptoms. If your hot flashes are unbearable, seek professional help.

Currently, as part of the federally funded research focused on women's health, the National Institutes of Health (NIH), Office of Alternative Medicine sponsors clinical trials at the Columbia University College of Physicians and Surgeons. They work to substantiate safety and effectiveness claims of many herbs and dietary supplements. The results of their research will help to establish quality and regulatory standards. In the meantime, you may wish to take your chances. Side effects are virtually nonexistent if you follow the instructions on the label.

There are some simple things that you can do to make your experience with hot flashes less troublesome. For instance, you can prepare for hot flashes or night sweats by dressing in layers and sleeping in the appropriate attire. Turn down the thermostat before retiring and have a pitcher of cool drinking water at your bedside. Keep in mind that the hormonal adjustment usually will take from 1 to 3 years and after that the hot flashes will subside. And as for the steps you took to deal with the problem (i.e., eliminate caffeine, alcohol, and nicotine), continue them. *The Change'll Do You Good.*

6

Vaginal Dryness/Atrophy

What's amiss I'll strive to mend,
And endure what can't be mended.
—Isaac Watts

❧

A S THE ESTROGEN LEVEL DECREASES, the genital area changes. The walls of the vagina become thinner and lose their elasticity. For women who experience vaginal dryness (sometimes called vaginal atrophy) sexual arousal no longer causes the same level of lubrication. Sexual intercourse can become painful. Susan remarked, "I'm to the point that I don't even want to have sex anymore!" Sexual activity may become painful and cause bleeding for some women. Although less than 20 percent of menopausal women experience vaginal dryness, most can alleviate discomfort with some simple behavioral changes. Serious problems require advice from a physician.

What you can do:

Let's start with what to avoid. Since vaginal dryness can cause pain and irritation, many women elect to refrain from sexual activity. This causes the problem to worsen creating a vicious circle. The more pain and/or irritation experienced, the less sexual activity, and with less activity, there is less natural lubrication. The reverse is also true. Your risk of vaginal dryness decreases with increased sexual activity. Just like the tissue in the rest of your body, if you don't use it, you'll lose it. For that reason, sexual activity can and should be considered a health behavior. That does not mean that you simply accept the potential discomfort. You may find over-the-counter products such as Astroglide and K-Y jelly useful for added lubrication. If the problem is severe and all else fails try estrogen in cream form. But before you do, read Chapter 34 on hormone replacement. Not having a partner is not necessarily an impediment to sexual activity. Although you may find sexual activity more satisfying with a partner, consider masturbation an option if you do not have a partner. Think of this behavior as forever. *The Change'll Do You Good.*

7.

OSTEOPOROSIS

There are no shortcuts to any place worth going.
—BEVERLY SILLS

☙

OSTEOPOROSIS IS A PREVENTABLE BONE DISEASE, common in aging, resulting from lack of sufficient calcium absorption in bone tissue. Prior to menopause, estrogen plays an important role in maintaining bone density in women by facilitating calcium absorption. With increasing age and diminished production of estrogen, the ability for bones to absorb calcium decreases, weakening the skeletal structure. Your bones become thin and brittle.

Risk Factors For Osteoporosis

You:

✴ have a relative with the disease

✴ have a small bone structure

✴ have low weight

✴ are Caucasian or Asian

✴ experienced early menopause (natural or surgical, prior to age 45)

✴ smoke cigarettes

✴ have a diet high in salt, protein, caffeine, alcohol

✴ have a diet low in calcium and/or vitamin D

✴ do not exercise regularly

✴ have or had an eating disorder

✴ take or have taken steroids

What you can do:

The National Osteoporosis Foundation recommends that you consider the following questions:

✴ Should I worry about preventing osteoporosis?

✴ How can I strengthen or preserve my bones?

✴ What type of exercise is best?

✴ How much calcium do I need, and what are the best sources of calcium?

✴ Should I have a bone mass measurement?

✴ How often should I have my bone mass measured?

✴ Do I need to consider medical treatment? If yes, what are the benefits and risks of these treatments?

I will attempt to guide you to find answers to those questions. Remember, osteoporosis sneaks up on you. Therefore, most women do not know that they have it. They usually discover it when they are in their 70s or 80s when they see a doctor for treatment of a fracture, usually as the result of a fall. At that juncture they are faced with an existing condition. You may be fortunate and still able to rebuild bone mass with the use of prescription drugs. For some that won't be the case. By then the progression of osteoporosis will have taken hold. If you are concerned because of your race, frame, build, and family history that you may be at risk for osteoporosis, you may want to begin monitoring your bone density. The ideal time to begin is before the onset of menopause.

Monitoring will supply you with an early warning system. A simple non-invasive test establishes a baseline for effective monitoring. Baseline tests ascertain your individual "normal" bone density level, the level you will seek to maintain. Bone density tests compare your bone density to that of a healthy young woman. The baseline approach allows you to compare your current bone density to your bone density level when the baseline test was taken. In other words, with the baseline approach, you measure actual changes in your bone density rather than measuring against statistical information.

In addition to monitoring your bone density you will need to make changes in your nutritional and exercise programs. *The Change'll Do You Good!* Let's explore each of these.

8.

Monitor Your Bone Mass

You can observe a lot just by watchin'.
—Yogi Berra

❦

If you are among the high-risk group talk to your doctor about osteoporosis. You can begin to assess your bone health with a baseline bone density measurement. Andrea (31) questioned, "My mother's sister has been diagnosed with osteoporosis, is it too early for me to get a baseline scan?" Linda had an early surgical menopause (30) and wondered the same thing. Now is the time for both of these young women to begin by getting a baseline scan. If three or more of the risk factors for osteoporosis apply to you, it is time for a baseline bone scan. Of course if you are already peri- or post-menopause, do it as soon as you can. The earlier you establish a baseline measure, the better.

The current test in use, DEXA (dual energy X-ray absorbtometry), is a painless noninvasive 20-minute procedure that measures hip and spine bone density. The computerized X-ray machine graphs bone density and compares your bone density to that of an average, healthy woman in the appropriate age range. That's why it is best to get your baseline DEXA as early as possible. If you establish a baseline when you are a healthy young woman, you will then be able to compare your DEXA later in life to your earlier scan.

DEXA can detect a loss of as little as one percent of bone mass from year to year. The cost of this test is $300 to $350 and can be requested through your personal physician or HMO. You can also directly order one yourself as you can with all of the baseline indicators. Once you start this program, you will have your own reading and can compare your later readings to your own baseline reading. You will be able to see how stable your bone mass is by comparing DEXA reports. I suggest that you keep a copy of your DEXA printout in your personal file for later comparison. In addition, after menopause, it's a good idea to repeat the screening every 3 to 5 years depending on your risk for osteoporosis.

Now that you know about baseline readings, use the same basic principal for mammogram screening. The American Cancer Society suggests that you start with a baseline mammogram in your late 30's or early 40's. As with the DEXA, your physician can refer you or you can directly order a mammogram yourself and ask for a copy for your personal file. That way, in the future, you will have a copy if the necessity to compare arises.

MENOPAUSE PREPARATION CHECKLIST

MAMMOGRAM

____ Baseline mammogram

    ____ Appointment time and date_____

    ____ Copy for personal file

____ Baseline DEXA - or other bone density measurement

    ____ Appointment time and date_____

    ____ Copy for personal file

9.

You Will Become What You Eat!

Destiny may shape our ends, but it gets
a lot of help from the food we eat.
—FANNY FERN

⚹

IMENTIONED EARLIER THAT OSTEOPOROSIS is preventable and it is. In part, exposure is beyond your control as certain groups are at greater risk. Women who are Asian or white, thin or small-boned, and/or drink more than two alcoholic drinks per day are at higher risk. Women who are African-American, overweight, and who exercise a lot are at less risk. In either category, there is still risk and DEXA will act as a gauge for your health behavior program. If you are losing bone mass, you will need to make adjustments in both your exercise and nutrition programs. The adjustments will be in the form of adding weights during regular exercise (see Chapter 20), and/or increasing calcium and vitamin D intake (see Chapter 29). And remember, the choices you make today will directly affect your future chances.

10.

REDUCE RISK OF
OSTEOPOROSIS AND
HEART DISEASE

Too often the great decisions are originated and given
form in bodies made up wholly of men,
or so completely dominated by them that
whatever of special value women have to offer
is shunted aside without expression.
—ELEANOR ROOSEVELT

❧

THERE ARE TWO GENERAL SCHOOLS OF THOUGHT in the critical arena of osteoporosis and heart disease. Some women choose to use prescription drugs in order to maintain estrogen at pre-menopausal levels to protect themselves from osteoporosis and heart disease. Others choose to increase their calcium, vitamin D intake, and to do exercise. Research has shown that adopting these dietary and exercise changes will decrease your chance of osteoporotic hip fractures. It is safe to say that research results on this very controversial topic emerge almost on a daily basis, sometimes raising more questions than they answer.

The National Institutes of Health (NIH) are trying to answer some of these questions through the Woman's Health Initiative, a collection of overlapping research studies. Cumulatively the 15-year project involves 164,500 women aged 50-79, the largest study of its kind in the world. The underlying goal of these studies is to understand what determines the health of post-menopausal women and to evaluate popular interventions. It will be a long time before we have the results of the initiative, but right now there is no question that lifestyle strongly influences risk for disease.

Since lifestyle evolves over time, modifying one's lifestyle is easier said than done. Your lifestyle results from an accumulation of your experiences throughout your life. It is a collection of habits, so to speak. During the first half of your life, you have little or no control over a large portion of your experiences. You cannot choose your family or the lifestyle to which they adhere. Yet your family, by the example it sets, establishes the course for many of your behaviors as you mature. Those behaviors that work well for you then become habits. The problem is that many of the behaviors that worked well for you in the past will not necessarily work well for you in the future. For instance, the petulance, sulkiness, and temper tantrums that got us what we wanted as children is detrimental behavior as adults.

At this time in your life, more than ever before, you have the ability to make lifestyle choices that will directly influence the quality of your lifestyle after menopause. Now, you no longer depend on your parents, you have made your decisions regarding children, and you generally understand your own limitations. There will never be a better time to get started. *The Change'll Do You Good!*

11.

IS MENOPAUSE SYNONYMOUS WITH OLD AGE?

The future has a way of arriving unannounced.
—GEORGE F. WILL

⚜

A S WE LOOK BACK AT HISTORY, we find that very little was known or said about menopause because as an event it was so rare. Very few women lived long enough to experience it. During the height of the Roman Empire (about 275 B.C.), for example, life expectancy for the average woman was 26 years. Therefore, any woman who experienced menopause was very old by ancient standards. Through the centuries physicians have concocted a variety of cures for the ailments that sometimes appeared around the time of menopause. In the 1600s and 1700s prescriptive remedies included such innovative and creative treatments as eating raw eggs or ground animal ovaries, to the old standby, bleeding by leeches.

Life expectancy slowly inched to the age of 49 by 1900. By then, women who reached menopause were not so rare but they were still few in total numbers and were seen as the elders of the community. Although there was no scientific basis, some in the medical community began to link emotional and mental stability with menopause. As yet, very little was known about menopause but its perceived negative effects were widely (and wildly) speculated on and those unsubstantiated speculations were accepted as fact. It's no wonder that historians considered menopause as the onset of old age. Of course, after you finish reading this book, you won't believe that anymore and *The Change'll Do You Good!*

12.

Myths of Menopause

Diseases desperate grown
By desperate appliances are relieved . . .
—William Shakespeare

⚜

In the late 1800s, in the Royal Edinburgh Asylum, 196 out of 228 cases of older women patients were labeled "involutional melancholia," the menopausal form of insanity. The accepted methods of treatment were like a page from the Spanish inquisition: ice water injected into the rectum, ice into the vagina, leeching of the labia and cervix. Sigmund Freud was of little help. He described menopausal women as "quarrelsome and obstinate, petty and stingy, and sadistic." During the 19th century in the United States, the removal of the ovaries was used as a treatment for insanity. Today, women are no longer institutionalized during menopause. However, enlightenment was slow to arrive. Even though no evidence links insanity in any way to menopause, as recently as 1980 "involutional melancholia" was still listed in the Diagnostic and Statistical Manual of Mental Disorders, a diagnostic tool used by psychiatrists. That means that as recently as 1980 it was still a valid psychiatric diagnosis.

The advent of antidepressants and tranquilizers in the 1950s provided a framework for prescriptive treatment of menopausal symptoms. Pharmaceutical companies mounted a vigorous campaign during the 1960s to promote psychotropic drugs for the treatment of menopausal symptoms.

Then the emphasis shifted from the mind to the body. Women were not insane, they had a disease. And, in fact, they had a disease that was curable with a product already on the shelf, synthetic estrogen.

As the old adage goes, give a problem to a carpenter and he will solve it with a hammer and a nail. . . . no matter what the problem is. Physicians, along with the pharmaceutical companies, solved the menopause problem with prescription drugs. There is no doubt that the notion of menopause as a deficiency disease has been very profitable for the pharmaceutical companies that produce and market synthetic estrogen. Women have bought right in to the theory because not only does it provide the "quick cure," but it also plays to our cultural idealization of youth. And once patients began estrogen therapy, many continued for the rest of their lives. The result: for years Premarin (synthetic estrogen) was the #1 selling prescription drug in the United States.

13.

THE TURNING POINT

You must do the things you think you cannot do.
—ELEANOR ROOSEVELT

U NTIL NOW MOST OF US HAVE THOUGHT the purpose of exercise was primarily to improve outward appearance, lose weight, etc. And since the human body, self-sufficient machine that it is, maintains itself to at least its basic level of necessity, most of us haven't had to think about our health very much. We have often heard that the most important thing is our health. Since our body doesn't ask for help until a critical need arises, we all tend to assume we will continue to enjoy the best of health.

In the case of women, nature provides the biological

strength during childbearing years to support the probable necessity to bear and rear children. Because our body does adjust to its perception of need, as we age and as our likelihood of child rearing diminishes, that same automatic biological system that kept us strong, now sees no need to continue to maintain the strong bone structure or cardiovascular system of our youth. In other words, nature keeps our bone structure strong so that we have the strength to rear children and once that time has passed it goes on to other tasks. How does nature maintain this strength? Through the production of estrogen. After menopause, when reproduction is no longer possible, it reduces the production of estrogen to meet the perceived need. Estrogen production doesn't stop; your body merely produces estrogen at a lower rate. As your body reduces estrogen production, you will need to make choices as to alternative steps to keep your bone structure strong. The actions you take now will determine your level of well-being in the future. Let's explore your options.

14.

READY OR NOT

. . . Age is opportunity no less
Than Youth itself, though in another dress.
—HENRY WADSWORTH LONGFELLOW

❧

EVERYTHING THAT IS WORTHWHILE takes time, effort and preparation. So plan ahead. Every successful person, no matter what field they have chosen, has put time and effort into preparing for their profession, craft or skill. Athletes and architects, doctors and draftsmen, teachers and truck drivers have all prepared and planned ahead. The time for you to prepare for life as an 80 or 90 year old is right now. The decisions you make today will relate directly to the quality of life you will enjoy in your later years. The plan you put in place today and the actions you deem necessary to execute that plan can never be made too soon. With determination and perseverance you can lay the foundation to be productive in your 70's, 80's, 90's and even 100 years old and beyond. It does take determination in the form of exercise and nutrition control to prevent the deterioration that naturally occurs in body tissue that goes unused and uncared for.

By her mid-30's, a women's body reaches its peak physical condition (measured by the level of bone density). From that point on there is a gradual deterioration. If you have taken action and have a DEXA prior to that time, you have a solid reference point. You can begin the steps necessary to prevent deterioration and you can measure your progress. If you are past your mid-30's, then start immediately. It is never too late. You have taken one positive step already by reading *The Change'll Do You Good* which will provide an outline of the "why" and "how" for you to have a positive influence on your aging process.

15.

LET'S GET STARTED

What we have to learn to do,
we learn by doing.
—ARISTOTLE

✤

W E ALL ARE ALREADY BEGINNING TO CHANGE the way we think of old age. Most notably we have moved the starting point. Not more than 20 years ago we thought of 50-year-old women as old ladies with blue-grey hair and little stamina or energy. How things can change! Today women like Diana Ross, Goldie Hawn, and Cher have had a dramatic influence on our image of the aging woman. This is not to say that you need to look like a movie star; although that may be nice. It is much more important that you remain functional for many years to come. Do not allow yourself to get sidetracked on the superficial. When you are 90 years old, it won't matter if your face has wrinkles or if your hair is grey for that matter. Whether or not you remain functional will matter greatly, however. By remaining functional you will be able to participate in interesting events, and therefore remain an interesting person.

What does it mean to remain functional? I have heard functional described as being able: to climb one flight of stairs, to stand up from a sitting position, to walk a city block. What ever happened to "able to leap tall buildings in a single bound?" On a more serious note, that minimal description may define functional for some but not for baby boomers, not for us. What may be more important is for you to think about what it means to you. What are the things you would like to continue to do throughout your life? Let's set some goals with real substance and meaning for you.

Try to visualize yourself functioning at the level you wish to maintain now and in the future. Is this what you really want? Fine tune the image until it represents 'you' in twenty, thirty years or more. Keep that image in your mind and keep yourself focused on that goal. Continually expand it! Visualize what you would be like in the year 2046. What would you like to be doing? If you would like to remain mobile, sharp-thinking, and productive, keep that clear picture in your mind. Use that picture as an incentive when you are having difficulty motivating yourself later on. Having that clear picture, that goal of who and how you can be will help keep you focused when interference arises in the future.

In order for you to remain functional for the next fifty years or more you must take action today. You must take steps to prepare yourself for that active, functional future. Preparation begins with the realization that this won't just happen. You will need a well-designed strategy of exercise and nutrition for your nonreproductive years. Such a program, if well designed, will meet the goal of maintaining body tissue and will lend itself to consistent repetition. In other words, the best program won't help if you don't do it. And before you begin any new exercise program, consult your physician. This is especially true if your lifestyle up to this time has been somewhat sedentary. And you know what? *The Change'll Do You Good!*

16.

3 x 20 = ONE HOUR PER WEEK

Nothing ever becomes real till it is experienced.
—JOHN KEATS

BEFORE YOU DECIDE YOU JUST DON'T have time (or desire) to exercise, let's look at the facts. The good news is that it doesn't take much! Studies have shown that:

20 minutes of weight-bearing exercise
that works up a sweat using your large muscles
three times per week

has proven beneficial in maintaining bone density, cardiovascular and respiratory health and a sense of well-being. What that means is twenty minutes of aerobics, jogging, fast walking, treadmill or any similar exercise that you choose, done three times per week will meet the criteria. You need to plan an activity that increases your heart rate enough for you to work up a sweat. Whichever you choose must be a weight-bearing exercise that utilizes your large muscles, those in your arms and legs.

Some additional tips: Start each exercise session with a 3 to 5 minute warmup designed to gradually work up a sweat. Begin your 20-minute session as soon as you begin to sweat. Once your routine is set, allow 30 minutes in your schedule. That will give you time for your warmup and you won't feel rushed. Then commit to do it 3 times each week without exception. In order to plant your workout firmly into your weekly schedule, formalize your commitment by writing the time and days that you choose on your calendar. Just a little over 1 hour per week of exercise and you are on your way to a better and healthier future. *The Change'll Do You Good.*

17.

Active Today — Active Tomorrow (And the Next Day!)

Well done is better than well said.
—Benjamin Franklin

✢

Now is the time to take a new look at your future. This is not an exercise program designed to make last year's clothes fit better. This is a program to provide you with a more productive life for years to come. You will need to make your exercise program a mandatory part of your life; a life-long activity just like brushing your teeth. That is why it is so important that you design or select a program that meets the criteria and that you will continue to do. You don't brush your teeth just when you feel like it; not if you want your teeth to be there as you age. The same is true of this exercise program. It is not an option; it is mandatory. And keep in mind that vision of yourself as you want to be many years from now. That should motivate you. And *The Change'll Do You Good.*

18.

WHAT'S A WOMAN TO DO?

Where to elect there is but one,
'Tis Hobson's choice—take that or none.
—THOMAS WARD

❧

ANY PROGRAM THAT MEETS THE CRITERIA and that you will do is the right program for you. Personally, I like step-aerobics for several reasons: (1) It doesn't require expensive equipment. You can purchase a step-aerobic package, including the bench and video, for under $70. And the only other thing you need is a good pair of shoes (See chapter 39 on shoes). (2) There is no wasted time. When you eliminate preparation and travel time you are down to a bare 30 minutes, three times a week. Even the busiest schedule can accommodate 30 minutes, three times a week! (3) Step-aerobic programs do not require special attire. Since you need not dress up for your workout, you save both time and money. You don't need to worry about your image or your appearance, because you can do step-aerobics at home. You don't even need clean socks. You can take care of them when you routinely do laundry. You can keep your sights on the important thing, to increase functioning in future years.

So you see, there is no room to give yourself an excuse for not exercising. If you don't feel well, you will feel better after you work out. Illness will only work as an excuse not to exercise when and if you are too ill to participate in any activities, even pleasurable ones. Other excuses (we all have them) such as, the weather is bad, my hair is a mess, etc, just won't fly since with step-aerobics you work out at home. You have no image to protect and preserve, just your bone structure, cardiovascular and respiratory systems. At the same time you will enhance your self-image as a high-functioning, active, and productive person in control of your own destiny.

19.

Exercising, The Fast and Easy Way

I wish to preach, not the doctrine of ignoble ease,
but the doctrine of the strenuous life.
—Theodore Roosevelt

⚘

There are many step-aerobic videos on the market today. If you already have one, start with that. If not, any one will do, since you will adapt the video you select to meet your program needs. Let's take a look at that in more detail. Most of the commercial videotapes designed for step-aerobic workouts start with a warmup and then run for about 40-45 minutes. Since you can meet the criteria by building up to and then maintaining a sweat for 20 minutes, you can start with a warmup of about 2 to 3 minutes. Then you can set a timer and after your warmup, workout for 20 minutes, and turn off the tape. Don't feel compelled to finish the tape; this is a life-long program and it is important that you stick with it. You will find that the entire workout, including warmup, will take less than 30 minutes.

20.

WEIGHT FOR WHAT?

Even when I was little, I was big.
—WILLIAM ("REFRIGERATOR") PERRY, CHICAGO BEARS

WHEN YOU STEP UP ON THE STEP-AEROBIC BENCH, you lift your body weight with the large muscles in your legs. That is a weight-bearing exercise. Therefore, you meet the criteria by lifting your body weight while keeping up a pace that causes you to sweat.

It may become necessary in some circumstances to increase that weight. For example, you may be at or under the median recommended weight found by the National Heart, Lung and Blood Institute guidelines for your height and build. Take a look at the Healthy Height and Weight chart and see where your weight falls. For women whose height falls between 4'10" to 6'4" this chart offers the weight range currently considered healthy. According to these guidelines, your weight must fall between the listed low and the listed high in order to be considered a healthy weight. For our purposes, look at the chart to see if your weight falls below the "Median" for your height.

HEALTHY WEIGHT CHART

Height	Low	Median	Highest
4'10"	91	105	119
4'11"	94	109	124
5'	97	112	128
5'1"	100	116	132
5'2"	104	120	136
5'3"	107	124	141
5'4"	110	128	145
5'5"	114	132	150
5'6"	117	136	155
5'7"	121	140	159
5'8"	125	144	164
5'9"	128	149	169
5'10"	132	153	174
5'11"	136	157	179
6'	140	162	184
6'1"	144	166	189
6'2"	148	171	194
6'3"	152	176	200
6'4"	156	180	205

If your weight falls below the median weight for your height and frame, you will add weights during your workout. Your risk level for osteoporosis is higher. How much weight should you add? The objective is to work out bearing up to 10 percent more than your actual weight in order to place a higher demand on your skeletal system. If your weight falls above the median healthy weight, you need not add additional weight.

By lifting more weight you will increase the demand on your bone structure. Don't rush it. If you need more weight start adding weight *after* your body has adjusted to your 20-minute workout. Don't add the weight all at once. Gradually increase weight by adding a weight belt and/or bar bells until you have worked up to the desired level.

Let's walk through the process. If, for example, your height is 5'4" and you weigh 120 pounds your weight falls below the median of 128. Your goal is to add up to an additional 12 pounds (10% of your body weight) during your workout. Remember, add the weight gradually, a combination of weight belt and bar bells will work well. Don't strain yourself. You have plenty of time, a lifetime for that matter, to add additional weight. Try talking during your workout. Never allow yourself to get out of breath. Only after you have mastered your regular 20-minute workout, add a four-pound weight belt. Take your time and allow yourself several workouts to adjust to the added weight. Then add two-pound bar bells. Again, there is no rush. It may take as long as a year to work up to what will become your regular workout routine.

If your weight falls between the median and the highest healthy weight for your height, there is no need for additional weight. Here is an instance where your weight works for you rather than against you.

If your weight falls above the highest healthy weight for your height then there is a different concern. In that case, an exercise program may put unusual strain on both the cardio-vascular system and the respiratory system and while the nutritional and exercise programs may assist in weight loss, a more cautious approach to exercise is essential. Keep in mind that this is not a weight reduction program; it is a program designed to provide us with the ability to function at a high level as we grow older.

21.

EXERCISE OPTIONS — NOT WHETHER, BUT WHAT

*The truth of the matter is that
you always know the right thing to do.
The hard part is doing it.*
—GENERAL H. NORMAN SCHWARZKOPF

༚

THE KIND OF EXERCISE YOU CHOOSE TO DO IS UNIMPORTANT. What is important is to do it regularly and that is what should govern your choice.

Fast walking, jogging, running, and aerobic dancing all qualify as weight-bearing exercises. Another possibility is stairs. If you live in a high-rise building, you may want to climb up and down several flights of stairs. Do any exercise you want as long as you sweat while exercising for 20 minutes consecutively, three times per week.

In addition to your formal program, add exercise to your daily living routine. Instead of parking in the nearest parking place, park in the furthest and walk to your destination. Instead of taking the elevator, take the stairs. Use your imagination to enhance your everyday life with exercise. And as always, *The Change'll Do You Good.*

22.

THE TIME OF YOUR LIFE

The wise, for sure, on exercise depend;
God never made his work for man to mend.
—JOHN DRYDEN

MAKE EXERCISE IMPORTANT TO YOU. Formalize your intent by writing your workout time on your calendar or schedule. You can exercise at any time of the day, but first thing in the morning usually works out the best. By making it your first order of business, exercise takes on a level of importance and it is easier to schedule. Just set your alarm 30 minutes earlier three times each week. You may find that Monday, Wednesday and Friday work well. A word of caution against selecting evenings for your workout. For one thing, you may be tired after your day of work and stress and it becomes easier to find reasons (activities other than exercise) to delay or defer it. Mornings also get the nod because exercise first thing sets the pace for your metabolism for that day and your metabolism is already slowing down due to menopause. Set the stage and save time by preparing in advance. If you do elect to use a step-aerobic program, gather your bench, video, shoes, and socks the night before. Rewind the video after each use so it will be ready for the next time. If you select another program, have your clothes and shoes set out the night before so that you will be ready to start bright and early the next day.

After your exercise routine, reward yourself. You deserve it. Take a refreshing shower with one of those great smelling gels. By making exercise your first and foremost priority, you will increase your self-esteem and start the day with a feeling of power and control. You will have a bounce in your step and a smile on your face. Yes, first priority means that you do your exercise routine before you eat or do anything else.

23.

So, You Hate to Exercise!

*'There's no use trying', she said:
'one can't believe impossible things.'
'I daresay you haven't had much
practice,' said the Queen. 'When I
was your age, I always did it for
half-an-hour a day. Why, sometimes
I've believed as many as six
impossible things before breakfast.'*
—Lewis Carroll

࿓

I'M CERTAIN YOU HAVE HEARD THIS BEFORE and you really don't want to hear it again. You're thinking "I've tried to exercise" and "I don't have the time for a special nutrition program." Or "I hate to exercise" and "I like junk food. I don't want to give it up!" Yes, you have heard it before and you will hear it again and again because it is true. But this book is about change and that doesn't mean just doing what you want to do. From what you have already read here, you know that your behavior must change if you are to remain functional and productive into your 80's, 90's and even 100 and beyond. As I researched for this book, I frantically looked for an easier way. Why? Because just like you I love junk food and I really, really don't like to exercise. After weighing all the alternatives, you can take my word for it. This is the easiest way.

We all know the advantages of regular exercise. And knowing that, it is still so hard to put our bodies into action. It's tough when the goal is short-term, such as trimming the excess fat to look good for our class reunion, or fitting into last year's swimwear for an upcoming cruise. And we know that when the goal is further away, a long-term gratification, the difficulty increases. It takes maturity, the ability to sacrifice now for future gain, to pull this off. You are investing time and effort now for a reward that will come in 30 years or more. Having your sights set firmly on your goal will help to motivate you. Keep that picture clear in your mind. The picture of you enjoying a happy, productive life in 2046.

You have heard many times that "You must like your exercise routine or you will not stick with it." Mary put it this way:

> I have tried all kinds of exercise. I'm good for about three weeks. After that for one reason or another I work out less and less until I'm back to not working out at all. I just can't seem to find an exercise routine that I like!

What if, after trying many exercise programs, you don't like any exercise routine? What if you are just like Mary (and many other women for that matter) and you do not like to exercise? Unfortunately liking it **DOES NOT MATTER.** That excuse will not fly. You still need to do it, even if you don't like it. You need to do it because research results show unequivocally that women who exercise regularly have significantly more bone density and lower incidents of heart disease than their less active counterparts. You need to do it because you want to remain functional for many years to come. You need to do it to keep yourself from becoming a vegetable in old age. So cheer up, *The Change'll Do You Good!*

24.

IS THE GLASS HALF EMPTY OR HALF FULL?

*The optimist proclaims that
we live in the best of all possible worlds;
and the pessimist fears this is true.*
—JAMES BRANCH CABELL

A S YOU SEE IN FIGURE 1, with a longer life span menstruation has become a smaller and smaller portion of ones life. Another fact that is less apparent, but important nonetheless, is when to prepare for productive later years. The answer is now. As you creep along the Life Line, you will find it much easier to prevent your body from deteriorating than to reverse it after the fact.

Life Line

_____ |___Menstruation_____ |_____ |...... |
Birth - 12 years   50.5 years   100 yrs - Death

Figure 1

Aging, another word for _living_, is an ongoing process. Take a look at Figure 1 above, Life Line. One thing about the menstruation phase that should jump out at you is that as your life span increases, menstruation becomes a smaller portion of your life. Most important of all, keep in mind that you can prevent enough natural aging deterioration of your mind and your body with regular exercise and close attention to your nutrition to remain functional.

25.

IS BONE MASS MORE IMPORTANT AFTER MENOPAUSE?

It is as painful perhaps to be awakened
from a vision as to be born.
—JAMES JOYCE

❧

BONE MASS IS NOT MORE IMPORTANT after menopause, maintaining it is more important after menopause. After menopause your body produces less of the hormone estrogen than it does prior to menopause. Thus, after menopause, you must consciously make an effort to maintain bone mass. By maintaining bone mass you will improve your posture and mobility as you age. In addition, you will decrease the likelihood of fracture and increase the likelihood of surviving an accident, a leading cause of death of those over age 65. You simply can not afford not to exercise. The evidence is in. If the goal is to remain functional in your later years, you are going to have to exercise, even if you don't like it.

If your lifestyle has not included regular exercise up to this stage of your life, check on your physical condition with your physician before you start. Then start gradually. Do not push yourself too hard in the beginning. It took you a lifetime to become the physical being you now are and you can't reverse it in a day. Take your time. Remember, remaining an active, vital, productive person is a life-long proposition. So take heart, *The Change'll Do You Good!*

EXERCISE CHECK LIST

____ Physical

    ____ Call for an appointment: date _____

                                   time _____

____ Set aside 30 minutes, 3 times a week, preferably first thing in the morning, Monday, Wednesday, and Friday

____ Mark your calendar / schedule with the times and dates selected

____ Choose an exercise that meets the criteria

____ Obtain supplies:

    ____ Bench

    ____ Video

    ____ Shoes

    ____ Other

____ Begin, gradually build up a routine that consists of:

    ____ 3-5 minute warmup

    ____ 20 minutes of sweat producing exercise

Remember, consistency is key. For this to work you must do it 3 times every week, no excuses.

26.

EIGHTY AND SHARP
AS A TACK

*Activity of the nervous system
improves the capacity for activity,
just as exercising a muscle makes it stronger.*
—DR. RALPH GERARD, NEUROPHYSIOLOGIST

჻

EXERCISE NOT ONLY HELPS TO PREVENT osteoporosis and heart disease, but also reduces nervousness, depression and/or mood swings as well. Although these are all symptoms commonly associated with menopause, it is wise to note that they do not originate with menopause. If you have experienced these symptoms earlier in life, you will probably continue to experience them during menopause.

Often what does happen is that these symptoms are exacerbated by negative life events, many of which happen to occur at the same time as menopause. As a result, many people have drawn the incorrect inference that because these behaviors became more noticeable at the time of menopause, they must be related to menopause. The fact is that reproductive biology cannot be blamed for general attitude, lifestyle, health, economic well-being, occupational status, or most other problems we may face at this particular time in life. However convenient it may be to blame menopause, it is not true.

Let's consider some circumstances that have an impact on lifestyle and often occur at the same time as menopause. Events such as divorce, children leaving home (sometimes referred to as launching), death of parents and other loved ones, and career changes can and often do coincide with the onset of menopause. All cause a high level of stress. Thus, any or all of these are far more likely to force symptoms of depression, nervousness, and/or mood swings to the forefront. And the good news is that exercise will help treat these symptoms no matter what their cause.

By now I hope that I have convinced you that exercising is a necessity if you wish to remain a healthy, active, and productive person beyond your reproductive years. This news is not as bad as it may first sound. A small amount of exercise goes a long way. The criteria I have outlined, three times per week, 20 minutes of load-bearing exercise, at a level that causes you to sweat, does serve as a minimum for a routine that will prevent loss of bone density and heart disease.

Don't be confused! This minimum will not cause weight loss or develop muscle tone. Those are problems with different solutions. And those are not problems that arise from menopause. An exercise program coupled with a well-devised nutritional program can most certainly bring about weight loss in an obese or seriously overweight person. That is not, however, our goal with the program I have outlined. I think it is critical to focus on that goal - preparing ourselves for a productive life into our 80's, 90's, and beyond. Commitment is the hardest part of beginning this or any other exercise program and that commitment is greatly strengthened by a clear focus.

For many women, the most difficult concept to embrace regarding menopause is not that reproduction is no longer possible or that menstruation has come to an end. Most women not only accept that aspect, they welcome that inevitability. Most difficult is the realization that exercise is no longer a choice they can make without serious consequences. Exercise has ceased to be an option; it has become mandatory! Once that reality is faced, the psychological commitment begins and you can develop a workout that will serve your needs and fit into your schedule. *The Change'll Do You Good!*

27.

PUMP IT UP — YOUR MEMORY THAT IS

Memory is a net;
one finds it full of fish when he takes it from the brook;
but a dozen miles of water
have run through it without sticking.
—OLIVER WENDELL HOLMES

❧

IS IT INEVITABLE THAT MY MEMORY WILL DETERIORATE? Maybe, but only to a certain degree. The stronger your memory to begin with, the stronger it will be later on. Memory, too, can be improved with stimulation. But first, let's review what we have been discussing. What we want to do is establish influence over the aging process. This is our goal. Doing this will give you a sense of power and naturally increase your sense of well-being. Taking steps in your 30's and 40's will give you the power to avoid some of the most common health problems after age 65, such as osteoporosis, falls, cognitive impairment, and depression. By taking control, you instill hope in yourself. You will know what to do, therefore, you will not think of yourself as helpless. You can take action. You have a plan and you follow it. Yes, left unchecked, bone mass declines after menopause as a result of normal decreasing hormonal changes, but you do something about it. You will successfully change your way of thinking and behaving by incorporating consistent exercise and healthy nutrition into your daily life. You are in control.

Regular weight-bearing exercise helps you to maintain bone mass and muscle tone, thus reducing the risk of falls and the resulting fractures, one of the most common health problems after age 65. This same exercise program, because it aids in bone strength and muscle tone, helps to maintain good posture through your later years, helping you to look and feel strong and energetic. In addition, your exercise and nutrition program will help to keep your blood circulating and your arteries flexible, thus reducing the risk of hypertension (high blood pressure). Strokes, which are related to high blood pressure, cause a large percentage of brain dysfunction in the elderly.

Let's return to preventing memory deterioration. Just like the rest of your body your brain needs exercise too to keep from deteriorating. You can sharpen your brain by continuing to learn. As we age we develop habits. This is nature's way of giving us a sense of security and well-being. We create through habit a circumstance that we are familiar with that allows us to

76

develop a comfort zone. That is why we take the same route to work each day and perform repetitive tasks. We are comfortable with them. They are in our comfort zone. The challenge now is to stop living entirely in that comfort zone. Take on the task of learning something new every day. Provide exercise for your brain by solving brain-teaser puzzles, or taking a new route to work. I could name endless possibilities, but that is really for you to do for yourself. Have fun exercising your brain. By learning something new every day you become a much more interesting person every day; the kind of person that draws others near. You will avoid becoming self-absorbed in medical problems as so many people over the age of 65 do. And again, *The Change'll Do You Good!*

28.

FIGHTING THE BLUES

*Nobody, as long as he moves about
among the chaotic currents of life,
is without trouble.*
—CARL JUNG

༯

DEPRESSION FEEDS ON THOUGHTS OF HOPELESSNESS and help-lessness. As an interesting, productive, socially active person, our chances of becoming depressed fall dramatically. Menopause does not cause depression. Chances of depression occurring during menopause are based on a history of depression, not on menopause. And since depression is rooted in hopelessness and helplessness, taking control of your aging process works to overcome the existing tendency for depression. Establishing a regular program that includes nutrition and exercise instills a sense of power. You will increase your sense of well-being, hopefulness, and control, thereby reducing depressive symptoms. There may be some who are so depressed that they lack the level of motivation necessary to make the necessary behavioral changes. In that case you should feel comfortable in consulting a psychologist for direction and assistance. Depression is treatable.

Even though depression is the most common psychiatric illness in the elderly, you are no more likely to be depressed in old age than in your earlier years. Such events as physical illness, medications and genetics commonly give rise to depression in the elderly. In addition, circumstances such as the mental strain emanating from the loss of a spouse, child, or other close relative, which cause depression in young and old alike, are more often encountered as we grow older. The simple reality is that those economic and health changes that would cause depression regardless of age occur more often in our later years.

In any case, depression is not a symptom of menopause and you will reduce your chances of experiencing depressive symptoms when you take control of your life by exerting a positive influence on your aging process.

BRAIN POWER CHECKLIST

_____ Learn something new every day

_____ Take a class

_____ Read a book, newspaper, magazine

_____ Read about ways to improve exercise and nutrition

_____ See new sights, vacation, etc.

_____ Take a new route to work

_____ Visit a museum, art exhibit

_____ Learn the rules of a sport

_____ Go to an opera, ballet, theater production
  _____ Learn about the production you will see

_____ Join/participate in a group that shares your interests

_____ Learn about a topic in depth, like "human origins"

_____ Learn any new skill, like sewing, painting, photography, etc.

_____ Solve brain-teaser puzzles, crosswords, etc.

29.

PEOPLE NEED PEOPLE

Man seeketh in society comfort, use, and protection.
—FRANCIS BACON

࿇

A S HUMANS WE ARE A SOCIAL SPECIES. We need social interaction. Yet we have seen many from earlier generations crawl into an inner shell as if to insulate themselves from an insensitive world. Whether as a result of illness, convenience, or fear, they stay within the confines of the most familiar, their homes. There they remain as if waiting for their time to end.

As the baby boom generation charts a new course, the challenge will be to keep from sliding on this slippery slope. Will we be able to keep from gradually isolating ourselves? Only with the commitment to expend direct energy to keep our social ties intact and maintain our comfort zones away from home.

We learned the importance of preserving our bodies and keeping our energy level up with consistent aerobic activity in Chapter 17. Not only will consistent aerobic activity serve to keep energy levels up during menopause but in later years as well. Developing and maintaining consistent aerobic exercise patterns will help to keep your energy level up as you age. Since you need to direct energy toward maintaining social contacts, your regular exercise program will help you to do that. Regular exercise will make you feel stimulated and propel you to activities outside of your home. But, exercise alone is not enough!

In Chapters 26, 27, and 28, the importance of keeping our brain in good working order was discussed. The ways to avoid depression, increase memory, and keep your brain sharp outlined in those chapters remain effective beyond menopause and throughout life. By keeping yourself healthy and alert you do your part to be an interesting and desirable social companion for others. So, make that extra effort. Be on guard. When you feel like closing everyone out, step out of your comfort zone and reach out to others. You are not the only one to benefit. Others that you reach out to will benefit as well. We are a social species and as such we need interaction with other human beings. Without that social interaction, we greatly reduce the quality of our lives.

30.

NUTRITION: A WAY OF LIFE

Tell me what you eat,
and I will tell you what you are.
—ANTHELME BRILLAT-SAVARIN

⚹

HOW CAN I PROTECT MYSELF against heart disease during and after menopause?

Prior to menopause your guardian angel (estrogen) reduced your risk of heart disease. Protected through young adulthood, you may have feasted on junk food, smoked cigarettes, and in general sowed your wild oats. All the while your greatest concern was 'How does my body look?' Now consider this radical thought — looks no longer take precedence. With menopause, priority shifts to 'How does my body work?' Bear in mind that when you are 90 or one hundred years old the critical focus will be on capability rather than on good looks. In any case, after menopause, in part due to the reduction in estrogen in your system, risk of heart disease among women equals that of men. Does that dictate estrogen replacement? Let's explore that question.

Along with exercise, you can strengthen your bone structure and cardiovascular system with proper nutrition. To build a strong cardiovascular system, it is critical to reduce plaque buildup and to keep your arteries flexible. To do this, along with regular exercise, you must reduce your overall fat consumption and increase the fiber content in your diet. The foundation of a healthy nutrition program begins with reducing calories that come from fat to 20 percent or less of your daily caloric intake.

Let's look at some basic facts to help you understand what this means to you in everyday situations. A gram of fat contains nine calories, a gram of carbohydrate or protein contains four calories, so reducing fat content will also reduce caloric intake. Do not confuse a healthy nutritious program with a weight reduction diet. Although you may lose weight while adhering to a healthy nutritional program, that is not the intent of the program. Obesity is not related to menopause and therefore is not addressed here. If obesity is a problem for you, you may desire professional help. When is it a problem? Take a look at the HEALTHY WEIGHT CHART on page 57. If you are over the maximum then you should take action to bring your weight into the range for your height. If you are at the top (within ten pounds) of the normal weight range for your height (as shown in the chart), your weight will help to maintain your bone density. Bones maintain their mass and strength to carry out tasks presented on a regular basis. Therefore, if you are at the top of the range (up to 10 pounds over), your bones will remain strong enough to carry your weight. If you are toward the bottom of the range, you don't need to gain weight, but will need to add weights to your exercise program. This will increase the demand on your bone structure and therefore provide the stress necessary for your bone structure to remain strong. And just like your exercise program, consider nutrition a life-long program.

Risk factors for cardiovascular disease:

Heredity
Age 51 and over
Hypertension (High Blood Pressure)
High blood cholesterol
Diabetes
Obesity
Cigarette smoking
Alcohol consumption

Look over the risk factors for cardiovascular disease. How many apply to you? Has a close relative had a heart attack before age 60? Have you checked your blood pressure lately? If three or more of the risk factors apply to you, your lifestyle habits may be increasing your vulnerability to heart disease. See your doctor for an evaluation and get advice on how you can improve your heart-health status. You can reduce a large portion of the risk factors with behavioral change. As with any prescription drug treatment, check out *Worst Pills Best Pills II* prior to beginning treatment. In addition, look for noninvasive options. For instance Anita shared:

Both of my parents had heart attacks before age sixty. My physician suggested a heart scan. It was a painless, noninvasive, procedure that gave a thorough representation of the current condition of my heart. My situation differs from that of my parents since I am very attentive to nutrition and exercise. Heredity, a very important risk factor, is the only one on the list that applies to me.

Primary ingredients to a healthy cardiovascular system:

Healthy nutritional program

Consistent aerobic exercise

Though more difficult than just popping a pill, you can build a healthy nutritional and consistent exercise program. It's a gradual process. Build it brick by brick, over time and get professional help if you need it.

As you begin to change to a healthy nutritional program, consider another test. If you haven't done so lately, have your cholesterol level checked. According to the American Heart Association, you should aim for a blood cholesterol level of 200 milligrams per deciliter (mg/dl) or less. Dietary fat consumption affects your cholesterol level. Avoid foods high in saturated fats, such as red meat, milk, eggs, cheese, all foods known to be high in animal fat. Instead choose fish, skinless poultry, skim milk, egg whites, and other nonfat dairy products. Remember, the foods you eat are the foods you and you alone choose.

In addition to paying attention to fat, think about fiber. A low fat, high fiber diet will reduce your chances of breast and colon cancer as well as heart disease. By increasing the fiber content in your diet, you will help to lower your cholesterol level. Remember that this program is designed to alter your diet and make it more healthy. That doesn't mean just eliminating items. It means replacing them with other tasty, but more healthy choices. One way to improve your eating habits is to look for the American Heart Association insignia on packaging.

Here are some guidelines. Your goal is to replace high animal fat in your diet with whole grains, beans, fruits, and vegetables. Limit red meat consumption to no more than two servings a week. However, there is no reason not to allow yourself to have foods that you really like. If you love Big Macs, for instance, have one. If you love chocolate, have some. The goal is not to deprive yourself, just limit the frequency and quantity of your consumption. One Big Mac during the month will not interfere with you nutritional plan, but one each day will. In between, try one of the low-fat counterparts like a veggie burger or turkey burger. After a while, you may find that you like those just as well.

And here's a good tip. Doctors and nutritionists alike recommend increased soy protein consumption during and after menopause. You can add soy protein to many dishes without interfering with the flavor. Be creative. Read more about the benefits of soy protein during and after menopause in *Dr. Susan Love's Hormone Book*, an excellent resource for the hormone decision as well.

Setting up and following a good nutrition program is challenging, but it will serve you for the rest of your long, productive life. And you will find that *The Change'll Do You Good.*

31.

CALCIUM: WHEN IS ENOUGH ENOUGH?

You never know what is enough
unless you know what is more than enough.
—WILLIAM BLAKE

L ET'S START WITH WHAT WE ARE LOOKING FOR. The recommended daily requirement of calcium increases for women during menopause from 1000 to 1500 milligrams per day (mg/pd). To be more specific, it is 1000 mg/pd prior to menopause, 1200 mg/pd during peri-menopause and 1500 mg/pd in the post-menopause phase. According to the book, *Worst Pills Best Pills II,*

> The best way to get calcium is to eat foods rich in
> it . . . In particular you can increase your calcium

intake by drinking milk and adding liquid or powdered milk to almost any cooked food. (Of course, you may want to use low-fat or nonfat milk to hold down your fat intake.) If you cannot get enough calcium from your diet, take a calcium supplement.

If you decide on a supplement, avoid those containing bonemeal and dolomite. Your bones will not absorb calcium as well from supplements containing those additives. Read the label to see how much elemental calcium the supplement contains. This portion is what counts as far as your body is concerned.

The foods you will want to include whenever possible include such standbys as:

Skim Milk	300 mg/cup)
Yogurt	415 mg/cup)
In addition, add to your list:	
Canned Salmon	300 mg/5 oz.
Canned Sardines	300 mg/1 1/2 oz
Shellfish - Clams, Oysters,	
Shrimp	30-35 mg/oz
Broccoli	195 mg/ 1 cup
Leafy green vegetables	93 mg/ 1/2 cup
Tofu	100 mg/2 .5x1"

Memorize the foods on this list and gravitate towards them. You make the choice whether you're in a grocery store or restaurant. When preparing food at home, increase the calcium content of any recipe by adding powdered skim milk. Develop the habit of reading the nutrition labels on packaging for the amount of calcium to be found in particular foods. Calcium is often listed as percent of the government daily requirement (1000 mg/pd), so you'll have to do the math but *The Change'll Do You Good.*

32.

WHAT ABOUT VITAMIN D?

Clay lies still, but blood's a rover;
Breath's a ware that will not keep.
Up, lad: when the journey's over
There'll be time enough to sleep.
—A. E. HOUSMAN

ﻋﻚ

VITAMIN D IS IMPORTANT BECAUSE IT HELPS your body to absorb calcium. The source of Vitamin D can be either dietary or exposure to the sun. Our goal is to fill the recommended requirement of 200 to 400 International Units (IUs) each day. Just like calcium, the best way to insure that you have enough Vitamin D is to eat foods that are rich in it. For instance, one cup of vitamin D fortified milk, contains 100 IU. And let's not forget the sun. Since exposure to the sun helps your body to produce Vitamin D, you may not want to avoid it. Of course we all know that exposure to the sun can be dangerous. We can have the best of both worlds if we use a sunscreen (15 SPF or higher) on all exposed skin all year round. Sunscreen will help to avoid damage to your skin from the sun and reduce risk of skin cancer while allowing you to benefit from the positive side of sunshine. *The Change'll Do You Good.*

The important thing is to take control of your nutritional intake by paying attention to the contents of the food you eat. If you owned an expensive car that called for high octane fuel, you would want to protect your investment so you wouldn't want to ruin the engine by putting low octane fuel in the gas tank. You probably know what happens when you put sugar into an automobile fuel tank. Adding anything but high octane fuel could be disastrous. You control your nutritional intake in the same way. Like precision equipment, your body is a highly complex system that requires particular nutritional ingredients in order to stay in top operating condition. And it is up to you to see that it receives what it needs.

33.

A Place In The Sun

I 'gin to be aweary of the sun.
—William Shakespeare

ℐ

To find a safe place in the sun we walk a fine line. We need vitamin D supplied by the sun, yet exposure to the sun's rays has been well established as a cause of skin cancer. Two forms of skin cancer, basil cell carcinoma and squamous cell carcinoma, may cause blemishes or deformities but can be cured if detected early. Melanoma, on the other hand, is often fatal and its incidence is rapidly increasing.

In the face of such danger some people still enter "tanning contests," and others place themselves in tanning booths that function sort of like a large toaster. Ironically, American culture depicts people with dark suntans as active, healthy, and attractive. Studies show that the same people who sunbathe to appear healthy are unlikely to engage in other health behaviors unrelated to appearance (like wearing a seat belt), they surround themselves with other sunbathers who reinforce their behavior, and they seem to be risktakers. Risktakers tend to be adventuresome without worrying about possible harm. Thus the studies concluded that sunbathers do not seek out healthy behaviors, but look for the appearance and social identity that indicate a relaxed and adventuresome approach to life.

Sunbathing is a complex health damaging behavior. Researchers suggest that understanding sunbathing behavior requires that one take into account a number of variables such as self-image, social influence, and personality. At first you may think it unusual to worry about suntanning but the same was true of cigarette smoking a generation ago. Today popular expectations are for a deep, dark, healthy tan just as movie stars glamorized cigarette smoking in the past. On a positive note, our culture has recently begun to shift away from and frown upon unhealthy behaviors like sunbathing and cigarette smoking.

At the other end of the spectrum, staying out of the sun completely isn't the answer either. Limited sun exposure provides essential vitamin D. So limit sun exposure and protect your skin by wearing protective clothing and sunscreens. Even in cold climates you risk skin cancer with over exposure to the sun. You can greatly reduce your risk by daily use of a moisturizer with a sunscreen rating of 15 or more on your face, regardless of the weather. If you plan to spend the day at the beach or on the golf course, use sunscreen on all exposed skin and replenish as necessary.

34.

STOP THE CRAVING

*I am very grateful to old age because it has
increased my desire for conversation and
lessened my desire for food and drink.*
—CICERO

IT IS IRRATIONAL TO THINK THAT YOU WILL have a healthy functional body 30, 40, or even 50 years from now if you continue to ingest large quantities of fat, over-processed foods, and junk food in general. If you are looking for an easy answer, stop. There isn't one. Providing suitable nutrition takes perseverance and determination. It is not easy and in fact in requires continuous effort. It is also a fact that you can develop a solid program one "bite" at a time. You already know the rules: Low fat, high fiber, proper vitamin and nutritional content. Now you need to start applying them. Begin with small steps. When choosing foods to eat, *always* look for the low-fat alternative. Small but consistent changes in your eating habits, such as using mustard instead of mayonnaise, will reduce fat. Choose whole wheat instead of white bread. And try low-fat desserts such as low-fat or fat-free yogurt instead of ice cream. You may find that you like the lower fat alternative as well or even better than your old stand-by.

The psychology of craving is that you crave the foods that you have developed a taste for. You've done this by eating those foods regularly and consistently. Now do the reverse. Stay away from that food or group of foods. For example, if you find yourself consuming too much sugar, take steps to greatly reduce your sugar consumption. Do this by keeping a written log. Mark your calendar each day that you are able to avoid sugar so that you can see your progress. After a few weeks, you will lose your craving for sugar. The same is true of your fat intake. If you stay away from Big Macs for a few weeks, you'll have fewer attacks. And I can promise you, *The Change'll Do You Good.*

NUTRITION CHECKLIST

___ Check your cholesterol level
    ___ Make an appointment

___ Reduce fat consumption to 20% calories from fat
    ___ Two or fewer servings of fried foods per week
    ___ Two or fewer servings of red meat per week
    ___ Switch to skim milk

___ Increase fiber
    ___ Increase grain, whole wheat bread, cereal
    ___ Increase vegetables
    ___ Increase fruit

___ Read food content labels on packaging

___ Look for the American Heart Association insignia on food packaging

___ Calcium mg/pd
    ___ 1000 pre-menopause
    ___ 1200 peri-menopause
    ___ 1500 post-menopause

___ Vitamin D, 400 - 600 IU/day

___ In order to reduce craving for a certain food, eliminate that food completely for a few weeks. Mark your calendar each day that you do not consume that food.

35.

Hormone Replacement Therapy

The patient, treated on the fashionable theory,
sometimes gets well in spite of the medicine.
—Thomas Jefferson

A S I SORTED THROUGH THE VAST ARRAY of reading materials on the subject of menopause, I came to realize that there was no clear-cut answer on hormone replacement therapy (HRT). While some hailed the advantages of HRT, others focused on the possible, unwanted side effects. And it is noteworthy that none of them recommended HRT across the board. The benefits that have been attributed (but not necessarily proven) to HRT include lower incidence of: hot flashes, vaginal dryness, heart disease, osteoporosis, nervousness, depression, and mood swings. In addition, there is some evidence of improved skin texture and in our youth-oriented society that cannot be overlooked. Many women report a greater sense of well-being. Based on this impressive list of benefits, women have turned to HRT in alarmingly high proportions. In fact, enough women have employed HRT to keep Premarin the number one best selling prescription drug in the United States.

How astonishing to say the least. I wondered why the number one selling drug in the United States is a drug that only a relative few would find useful to treat their symptoms. Yes, one would expect doctors to prescribe estrogen for women at menopause to treat symptoms such as vaginal dryness and hot flashes. But those symptoms arise in only a very small percentage of the cases. In fact, the evidence is that only about 5 percent of menopausal women experience these symptoms to the extent that warrants prescription treatment. So again the question arises, Why so many HRT prescriptions?

Some adopt the theory that HRT will reduce the incidence of heart disease and should be taken for life. While it is an optimistic and hopeful view, at this point in time, there is no conclusive evidence to that effect. Doesn't it make sense to also consider the possible side effects before embarking on HRT? *Worst Pills Best Pills II*, published by Ralph Nader's *Public Citizen Health Research Group*, a publication not related to or funded by a pharmaceutical company, described the possible results in the following warning:

> Using estrogens increases your risk of endometrial cancer (cancer of the lining of the uterus) by 6 to 8 times. This cancer can be cured by surgery only if it is detected early through a special examination

called an endometrial biopsy, and such biopsies are usually done only when a woman is bleeding abnormally. Taking estrogen has also been linked to breast cancer in both men and women. The risk is higher for women who take higher doses or who have used estrogen longer. Experts from the National Cancer Institute and from other countries state that 'the prolonged use of estrogens at the time of menopause may increase the risk of breast cancer by 50% after a 5 to 10 year interval.' (p.648)

Some physicians combine estrogen with progestin to decrease the chance of endometrial cancer. Progestin causes the shedding of the lining of the uterus. As a result, a woman taking progestin may bleed every month even after she has passed menopause. For most, this is not a pleasant thought. Many women consider the absence of bleeding after menopause a relief. They welcome the relief from sanitary napkins and tampons, but with progestin, bleeding (and the need for sanitary napkins or tampons) continues. Of Progestin, *Worst Pills Best Pills II* says:

> Progestin has been associated with blood clots, strokes, and blindness in women. The drug causes breast and uterine cancer when administered in laboratory mammals, and researchers are investigating whether it causes breast cancer in women by itself or further increases the risk of breast cancer when used with estrogen. (p.653)

The authors recommend limited use of no more than six to twelve months for these synthetic hormones. I should mention that I choose to quote *Worst Pills Best Pills II* because it is the result of work done by a group of doctors not affiliated with a pharmaceutical company. I found that most research published on this topic is sponsored by the pharmaceutical companies and, at best, that presents a conflict of interest. The analogy of the fox in the chicken coop comes to mind.

Yes, estrogen may decrease the incidence of osteoporosis — but at what cost? There is no clear evidence and certainly no guarantee that taking it will keep you from getting osteoporosis. However, there is clear evidence that estrogen is *not* effective for treating nervousness, depression and/or mood swings. Before making the HRT decision, consider both the results you want and the serious risks associated with it. Then remember you can achieve the desired results by changing your behavior as well, and without dangerous side effects. And guess what? *The Change'll Do You Good.*

36.

Alcohol — Three Cheers For The Designated Driver

What's drinking? A mere pause from thinking!
—Byron

T HE USE OF ALCOHOL (AND NICOTINE AND CAFFEINE) is woven into our culture. For many in our culture, it is hard to imagine going to a party or out to dinner (any social event for that matter) without alcohol consumption. Research on the use of alcohol has vacillated from positive to negative results. At the time of this writing, it is no surprise that moderation is recommended. What does that mean? No study condones more than two glasses of wine or two beers per day and none suggest the consumption of hard liquor. Studies show that drinking patterns change with age. The highest rate of consumption occurs between the ages of 21 and 34 years, with only two percent of women over age 65 considered heavy drinkers. So there seems to be a natural progression to consuming less alcohol as one ages and that is a good trend to follow.

Keep in mind that aside from the internal, physical dangers such as brain damage and liver disease, alcohol increases your risk for falls, fractures, and head trauma. Alcohol, a central nervous system depressant, disrupts thought, judgement and restraint, voluntary actions become clumsy, and affects emotional behavior.

In social situations, you may feel pressure to consume alcohol. Just like old times! Peer pressure is always with us. Here you have an advantage: you have experience with peer pressure and independent thinking comes more easily with age. You have reached a level of maturity that gives you the strength and confidence to fight off peer pressure. Plan ahead for those social situations at which you will usually consume alcohol. If, for instance, you know you will be in a bar, plan what you will order before you go into the bar. You make the choice as to what you will drink and your choices include soft drinks, iced tea and sparkling water instead of alcoholic beverages. Don't deprive yourself. You can still have a couple of glasses of wine or beer with dinner, just don't overdo it. *The Change'll Do You Good.*

37.

NICOTINE — WE'VE COME A LONG WAY

*O God, that men should put an enemy
in their mouths to steal away their brains!*
—WILLIAM SHAKESPEARE

❧

NICOTINE IS A DIFFICULT ADDICTION TO KICK. Some say the most difficult. One reason it is so difficult is that we weave our habits into our environment. As society accepts smoking in less and less of our environment, we have more and more encouragement to quit. As difficult as it is to quit, roughly forty million Americans have quit since the Surgeon General's warning in 1964. If you haven't quit smoking by now, you may consider yourself a "hard-core smoker." By this I mean that you have been able to successfully combat the tremendous societal pressure to quit.

Cigarette smoking satisfies different needs for different people. For many of us, it helped us to separate and individuate from our parents when we were adolescents. Our cigarette smoking behavior was something our parents could not control. It was something that aligned us on a united front with our peers. My parents were extremely wise. They knew that cigarette smoking was a health hazard even before the official announcement from the Surgeon General. Their warnings only verified that cigarette smoking separated me from them and that I was in control of my behavior, not them.

Whatever the reason that you smoke, whatever need the behavior satisfies, if you have attempted to quit in the past and have been unable to do so, get professional help. Find out what needs you satisfy with cigarette smoking behavior and how you can satisfy those needs with less danger to your health. It is irrational to think that quitting a behavior that you have participated in for many years will be easy. You must accept that you are in for a very difficult task. You can find a way if you are persistent and determined enough. Keep that picture of yourself years from now healthy and active in your mind. It will help to motivate you. Remember, if you are interested in staying functional throughout your life you must change your behavior and *The Change'll Do You Good.*

38.

CAFFEINE — STOP THE JITTERS

Throw physic to the dogs;
I'll none of it.
—WILLIAM SHAKESPEARE

❧

CAFFEINE, A STIMULANT SUBSTANCE found in coffee, tea, cocoa, cola, and other soft drinks, in some cold remedies, and in some diet pills, acts to increase metabolism, body temperature and blood pressure. Caffeine use may result in hand tremors, diminished appetite, and, most familiar of all, sleeplessness. Since candy and soft drinks contain caffeine, addiction can begin early in life.

How much caffeine are we exposed to? Some examples:

Coffee contains 100 - 150 mg. of caffeine per cup, cola drinks contain 25-55 mg. per glass, and a chocolate bar contains up to 25 mg. Learn to read the labels, especially on soft drinks. Surprisingly, even some non-colas contain high amounts of caffeine. As with any addiction, abstinence is difficult, yet attainable if you are highly motivated. Caffeine withdrawal symptoms usually last no more than four to five days. Detoxify your body gradually. Begin by substituting caffeinated soft drinks and coffee with those without caffeine.

Alcohol, nicotine, and caffeine play a major role in the frequency and intensity of hot flashes. If you are experiencing hot flashes, eliminate your intake of these drugs. Record your efforts in a daily log. The ability to see your progress will help to motivate you to continue. With persistence and determination you can greatly reduce or eliminate these drugs entirely and *The Change'll Do You Good.*

39.

NO SMALL FEAT

Somebody said that it couldn't be done,
But he with a chuckle replied
That "maybe it couldn't," but he would be one
Who wouldn't say so till he'd tried.
So he buckled right in with the trace of a grin
On his face. If he worried he hid it.
He started to sing as he tackled the thing
That couldn't be done, and he did it.
—EDGAR A. GUEST

༄

THROUGHOUT A LIFETIME, ON AVERAGE, you will walk 100 thousand miles, the equivalent of four times around the earth. Frequently we squeeze our feet into unsuitable footwear which has damaging effects on the entire body. Not surprisingly, as you pinch your feet into ill-fitting shoes, you walk around with a grimace rather than a smile on your face. You become irritable and often avoid walking all together. Let's face it, our world seldom offers the opportunity to walk comfortably on smooth surfaces. More likely, we walk on concrete, asphalt, and stone resulting in strain on our entire body. Knees, hips, and spine literally take a beating.

In view of these circumstances, one can easily see how before long, walking can become troublesome. Many, both young and old, avoid walking at all costs prefering to use public transportation or drive even the shortest distances. Yet, we know that if we wish to remain functional throughout our lives, our fate lies in our ability to remain mobile. Think for a moment of the image that you have of yourself as a functional 90 or 100 year old. One of the most important aspects of remaining functional is your mobility. Mobility, clarity of thought, and good general health will provide the foundation of an interesting and exciting life later on.

In fact, we give little thought to the importance of our feet. All through our lives we have taken them for granted. Often they hurt after a long day of work, but the next day they seem fine and we start all over again. Most often unsuitable footwear causes aching feet and poorly fitted shoes or high heels can lead to back pain, poor blood circulation and even headaches. In addition, inadequate footwear has a negative impact on posture and balance.

So why do we all continue to abuse our feet? One reason is that we were never really taught the importance of feet. As children our parents were more interested in teaching us the importance of our eyes. Hence, how many times have you heard that infamous "You could take an eye out like that!" Nevertheless, the only emphasis on feet focused on fashion. As a consequence, most of us have ignored the healthfulness of our feet.

What To Do:

As a person who takes their health seriously, begin by regularly giving some thought to your feet. The most important aspect of good foot health is properly fitted footwear. Women's shoe sizes increase with age. Hence, measure your feet when purchasing shoes. Buy comfortable shoes in the size that your foot measures. If it has been more than a couple of years since you've measured your feet, you may be surprised! Find shoes in a size and style that allow you to wiggle your toes. For the well-being of your entire body, fit your feet with high quality functional footwear.

Look for shoe styles suitable for the activity that you have in mind. Erroneously, athletic shoes represent the quintessential comfort shoe to many. In other words, running shoes are not the best for walking and vice versa. For walking, invest in a pair of high quality walking shoes, they will prove well worth it. Though expensive, they last a long time. Look for brands expressly offering footwear designed for optimal walking comfort. Once you have the right walking shoes, walk often and enjoy it.

You say, "But I like high heels, they make me feel dressed up, sexy, and taller!" You can still wear them and there is no need to deprive yourself. Simply limit your wear to occasions that will not require standing or walking to a great extent. Look for shoes with a heal height no higher than two inches and heal width the same from top to bottom. The new wider, more squared toe box doesn't squeeze toes as much. Most importantly, think of your feet as the foundation of your mobility. Without strong healthy feet, confinement of some sort is inevitable. Many women have already changed their view of shoes. It isn't unusual to see women in business suits wearing athletic shoes. As you pay more attention to the health and comfort of your feet, you will find yourself opting to walk more often and *The Change'll Do You Good!*

40.

IT'S PURE SEX

*Is it not strange that desire should
so many years outlive performance?*
—WILLIAM SHAKESPEARE

꙳

AS WOMEN OF THE BABY BOOM GENERATION, sexually, we went from oppression to liberation and back to conservatism. In the 1950's, we dared not speak of sex. It was truly a man's world. Men flaunted their sexual prowess while women were shamed for even the smallest interest. Those who became pregnant were shunned by society. Many were hidden away to avoid embarrassment for the family. The children were placed for adoption, while the mother was not afforded as much as a glance at her new offspring. Abortions took place illegally, in back rooms, and only to those with means.

All this came to a screeching halt in the 1960's. The equal rights movement (ERA) began the backlash. First bra burning, and then *Roe v. Wade*. Women wanted sexual freedom. Birth control positioned women on equal footing with men. Now women too could indulge in sexual activities without fear of pregnancy. College dorms became coed. Leaders of the ERA movement fought for a constitutional amendment. They sought equality for women in the workplace and in the military.

Those against the amendment claimed it wasn't necessary, that the Constitution already provided equal rights for women. They held tightly to the ideal of women as the weaker sex. In their view, women had their place as mothers, teachers, nurses, etc. After all, where would the line be drawn? It was their fear that women would be forced to the military draft and eventually to the battle front. ERA, never able to muster the support to pass, fell by the wayside.

In the 1970s, in the wake of ERA, compromise lead to new freedom for women. Women enjoyed their newfound freedom in the workplace, in the military, and yes, sexual freedom too. Though no longer shunned for sexual promiscuity, many women found that sex without emotional attachment left them with an empty feeling. Fast flings and one-night stands initially appeared as a fun and exciting way to experience sex, but turned out to be a barren wasteland of unrealized affection.

Most women were left feeling emotionally drained. General disenchantment with sexual openness grew among women with the advent of AIDS in the early 1980s. Both men and women began to reconsider the prudence of promiscuous sexual behavior. In the 1990s, the government sponsored controversial yet expansive AIDS education programs. As a result, sexual restrictions arose that were self-imposed rather than societal in nature.

Menopause, a double-edged sword for sexual activity, reduces inhibition even further. Menopause negates the need for birth control, yet for many women, vaginal atrophy substantially diminishes their ability to enjoy sex (see Chapter 6). As a result, mistakenly, many believe that sexual desire wanes as we age. We know that is incorrect because we see that AIDS incidence in the population of those over 65 years of age is rapidly increasing. Initially that population was ignored. It was thought that preventive measures were not necessary for older Americans since, it was believed that they were inactive. That thinking has been proven wrong. Research shows that people are sexually active all of their lives. Your sexual experience as you age will depend largely on your sexual experience thus far. It is an individual thing. You have developed your own meaning of sex through the events of earlier life. If you have enjoyed an active sex life throughout young adulthood, you will continue to be sexually active later in life. Your only restrictions are those you impose upon yourself. You determine your sexual activity after menopause by the level of importance you place on sex.

Human sexuality reaches far greater meaning than just reproduction, thus menopause does not reduce the desire for sex. Depending on its meaning to you, sex can provide intimacy, tension reduction, and a general sense of well-being all through your life. Recently different definitions have been offered as to what constitutes sex. For our purposes here any activity that involves touching or stimulating of ones genitals can be considered sex. Touching may be with or without a partner. This includes fondling, masturbation, oral sex, as well as intercourse, or sexual activity within your comfort zone that brings gratification.

Sexual enjoyment requires muscle tone. Atrophy (muscle deterioration) occurs in the walls of the vagina for the same reason it occurs in other muscles of the body; lack of use. In order to retain muscle tone operate those muscles! Yes, sexual activity generates sexual activity. With frequent stimulation your body releases a lubricant to facilitate intercourse. After menopause you may find a synthetic lubricant such as KY Jelly or Astroglide useful. Don't be afraid to experiment. Though I do not endorse or encourage promiscuity, your ancestors and counterparts fought long and hard for sexual freedom. Now only you provide and enforce the restraints that apply to you.

Sexual contentment provides more than physical enjoyment. It enhances self-image and gives one a sense of well-being. If you have a partner, so much the better. Nothing creates a sense of intimacy between two human beings as sex does. If you do not have a partner, you can still experience the joy of sex through masturbation. Enjoy sex regularly, at least three times a week, to keep yourself feeling confident, healthy, and youthful.

41.

PUT SOME TEETH INTO IT

*Every tooth in a man's head
is more valuable to him than a diamond.*
—CERVANTES

༄

NO DISCUSSION OF LIVING A LONG AND HAPPY LIFE would be complete without touching on the topic of dental care. Excellent overall health includes excellent oral health. Earlier generations were not overly concerned with their teeth and gums. Thus, many of our parents and grandparents replaced their teeth with dentures. Back then the focal point was not maintaining good oral health in order to enjoy a better quality of life in later years. Instead the tasks of daily life held their interest. Fortunately, modern technology allows most of us spend less time maintaining our home and clothing or preparing food than previous generations did. Since we will live longer it is important that we recognize the trade off and spend more time than previous generations on physical fitness. For the first time we know that we will live longer than any generation has in the past and we have the foresight to prepare ourselves for those later years. That includes attention to our dental health. Moreover technology has rapidly reduced discomfort related to dental work and many employers and health care insurance companies offer dental benefits.

All of those reasons not withstanding, many of us do not take the time for regular dental care. Dina Provenzano, D.D.S. has worked with geriatric populations as part of the Northwestern University Dental School geriatric program. When asked to describe an overall plan to avoid dental problems and tooth loss for women facing menopause Dr. Provenzano said:

> Most dental disease diagnosed in the forth and fifth decades is a result of gum disease. People think that just because cavities no longer pose a problem they do not need regular dental care. However, as a result of receding gums, root decay often becomes a serious problem. Fortunately, if caught early enough, gum disease can be treated. That is why it is important for people over forty to have regular check-ups. I recommend that all people including those over age forty have their teeth checked and cleaned twice a year. Most dental disease can be readily addressed if diagnosed early and monitored by a dental professional regularly.

When asked about daily care between check-ups, she said:

> The daily fight is against plaque buildup. It forms

on tooth surfaces continuously. After twenty-four hours if it is not removed, it builds up and turns to tartar. At this stage it becomes dangerous to gums and to the integrity of the teeth. Plaque is made up of bacteria that find their strength in numbers. They group together in between the teeth and below the gum line. After several days inflammation and bleeding of the gums is found as a result of gum infection and response to the foreign plaque. To stay healthy, reduce the number of plaque bacteria on a daily basis. That is what proper flossing and brushing does.

We can conclude that it is important to floss once and brush your teeth ideally twice but at least once within every twenty-four hour period. Preventive dental care can become a healthy habit that will be rewarded by a lifetime of whiter, healthier teeth and pain-free gums, not to mention beautiful smiles. It requires discipline at first, but you will find adopting good oral hygiene relatively easy to do. It is "relatively" easy to do because even minor behavior changes, such as adding two minutes of tooth flossing to your routine, can be very difficult. You can make the behavior change more easily by thinking of flossing and brushing as a regular part of your daily hygiene routine rather than something extra. Initially, seeing immediate visible results in a written log may help you to get started. When after extraordinary determination and perseverance you can not bring about the change, it is time for professional help.

42.

IT ALL ADDS UP

Nothing is ended with honour
which does not conclude better than it began.
—SAMUEL JOHNSON

❧

No, MENOPAUSE WILL NOT BE WHAT IT FORMERLY WAS. The baby boomers have changed that. Only time will tell what their experience will be. We know for sure that they will live longer than any of their predecessors. Besides, for the first time they will have the opportunity to prepare for life at 80, 90, or over one hundred years. As a case in point, Cynthia quoted her one hundred and two year old grandmother: "If I knew I would live this long, I would have taken better care of myself."

Maybe if her invalid grandmother had more time when she was young to engage in more health behaviors, she would have maintained her mobility. Her quote starts with the words "If I knew. . ." That's the difference. The baby boomers do know. You know. It is up to you to do something about it. The quality of your life in years to come depends largely on the actions you take now.

It's a big responsibility, living so long. There's so much to do. It may seem overwhelming at first but you can get it all under control. If you feel that you do not have the time or the energy to do all of these things, consider your individual situation. For instance, Nancy (36) chided, "In my busy life, between my two preschoolers and my career I have little time to spend with my husband. I don't have time to exercise." For Nancy, the exercise program was not immediately critical. Considering her age and activity level, she can put off beginning a regular exercise program until some time in the future. In her case, it would be more meaningful to:

> Begin with a baseline bone scan and mammogram and keep a copy of each in her personal file for later comparison.

> Focus on those things that do fit into her schedule now, such as attention to nutrition, dental care, everyday health behaviors, etc. At 36, Nancy has plenty of time to begin a consistent exercise program when her family demands less of her time.

> Periodically go over the checklists at the end of the chapters to increase your awareness. As you integrate each health behavior, go back and make a check mark in the provided space.

It may seem overwhelming at first. This quick list will help to raise your awareness of the health behaviors outlined in this book:

⚹ Keep your bone structure strong by monitoring your bone mass.

⚹ If you are over 50 years of age, have a mammogram once a year as the American Cancer Society recommends.

⚹ Pay special attention to nutrition.
Look for low fat alternatives.
Increase fiber, calcium and vitamin D.

⚹ Sweat-producing exercise, twenty minutes, three times a week.

⚹ Assess all of your options before taking any drugs (HRT, etc.).

⚹ Floss and brush your teeth daily and get a check-up every six months.

⚹ Everyday health behaviors:
Choose the furthest parking place instead of the nearest.
Take the stairs instead of the elevator, etc.
Wear seat belts when driving or riding in a car.

⚹ Perceive menopause as a liberating, self-empowering time of your life.

⚹ Step out of your comfort zone to present yourself with new stimulating material.

⚹ Make an effort to interact with others regularly.

⚹ Avoid unnecessary drugs: alcohol, nicotine, and caffeine.

⚹ Wear comfortable shoes that fit your feet and allow room for your toes to move freely.

⚹ Use sunscreen rated 15 or higher on skin exposed to the sun.

⚹ Engage in regular sexual activity.

Some of these you already do. The others can be incorporated into your lifestyle with determined commitment. Allow yourself to make behavior changes one step at a time. As for this list, the whole far outweighs the sum of the parts. With each incremental step you make a geometric progression toward your goal. I do not present this as a comprehensive list, but merely a starting point. Continue to watch for research results of the Women's Health Initiative. Data collected from these and other studies will guide you to expand the list through the coming years. For in-depth coverage of the material touched upon in this book, see the recommended reading list in Appendix 1. Indeed, expanding your knowledge and awareness will increase your chances of living a healthier, longer, thus happier life.

Aside from knowledge and awareness, use your common sense. You developed a goal for remaining functional in later years. Keep that clearly in the forefront of your mind and your unhealthy behaviors of the past will soon fall by the wayside. With your new health behaviors you can look forward to the baby boom generation centennial in 2046!

APPENDIX 1

Read More About It

Pharmaceutical Reference

Wolfe, Sidney M. & Hope, Rose-Ellen. *Worst Pills Best Pills II.* Washington, DC: Public Citizen Health Research Group, 1993. *Describes usage, side effects, and safer alternatives of pills.*

Hormone Replacement Therapy

Love, Susan M. & Lindsey, Karen. *Dr. Susan Love's Hormone Book.* New York: Random House, 1997. *Overview of menopause answering questions about HRT from a medical perspective.*

Kamen, Betty. *Hormone Replacement Therapy Yes or No?* Novato, CA: Nutrition Encounter, Inc., 1993. *Nutritional alternatives to HRT.*

Comprehensive

Henkel, Gretchen. *The Menopause Sourcebook.* Los Angeles: Lowell House, 1994. *Information on every aspect of menopause.*

General Overview

Furman, C. Sue. *Turning Point.* New York: Oxford University Press, 1995. *Practical implications of menopause.*

Lark, Susan M. *The Menopause Self Help Book.* Berkeley, CA: Celestialarts, 1990. *Guide in workbook form.*

Osteoporosis

Bonnick, Sidney Lou. *The Osteoporosis Hand Book, Every Woman's Guide to Prevention and Treatment.* Dallas TX: Taylor Publications, 1997.

Alternative Medicine

Duke, J.A. *The Green Pharmacy.* Emmaus, PA: The Rodale Press, 1997.

CRITICAL CONCEPTS

Aging - Living.

Alcohol, nicotine, caffeine - socially acceptable drugs.

Alternative medicine - The practice of using dietary supplements, herbs, vitamins/minerals and mind/body interventions (i.e., acupuncture), to remedy a condition.

Baby boomers - The generation born between 1946 and 1964.

Cardiovascular disease - Irregularities in the vascular system, including the heart, that lead to malfunction.

Critical concepts - Short definitions of terms as used in this book.

DEXA - A non-invasive procedure used to measure hip and spine bone density.

Disease model - This model views problems from a medical perspective. The recipient is neither responsible for the disease nor the cure. The individual must rely on a medical expert to solve problems usually with perscriptive medicine or other invasive means.

Functional - Ability to carry out daily living tasks.

Health behaviors - Things you do to remain healthy (i.e. wear seat belts, etc.)

Hormone - A substance produced by one body tissue and conveyed by the bloodstream to effect another body tissue. Estrogen, a hormone produced chiefly by the ovaries, regulates certain female reproductive functions and maintains secondary sex characteristics.

HRT - Synthetic hormones, taken in pill form or dermatological patch, that must be prescribed by a physician.

Hot flash - Feeling very warm to intense heat, usually lasting 2-3 minutes.

Irrational thought patterns - Thoughts that lead to irrational behavior (i.e., "I can maintain mobility indefinitely without exercise).

Memory - Function of the brain that is enhanced by stimulation.

Menopause - The end of menstrual bleeding.

Minimum aerobic exercise - Twenty minutes, sweat producing exercise, three times a week.

NIH - Research agency sponsored by the federal government.

Osteoporosis - A preventable bone disease, common in aging, thought to be triggered by reduced estrogen levels.

Peri-menopause - The time, when hormone levels decrease enough to cause changes in the menstrual cycle, between normal menstrual cycle and post-menopause.

Post-menopause - Menstrual bleeding has ceased for twelve months or more.

Psychotropic drugs - Drugs used to alter the chemistry of the brain.

Sunscreen - Lotion or cream containing chemicals, measured by SPF, that block ultraviolet rays.

Symptoms of menopause - Hot flashes, night sweats, and vaginal dryness or atrophy.

The blues - Feeling sad, worthless, hopeless, and/or helpless, inability to take pleasure in daily activities, feeling lethargic and fatigued, recurrent thoughts, inability to concentrate, sleep and/or weight disturbance, to the extent that these feelings interfere with daily living.

Vaginal dryness/atrophy - Degeneration of vaginal wall tissue and loss of lubricants that may cause pain during sexual activity.

Women's Health Initiative - A collection of research studies, funded by the federal government, devoted to women's health.

ORDER INFORMATION

To order additional copies of *The Change'll Do You Good* forward the following information to:

DCS Publishing
33 West Huron, #809
Chicago, IL 60610

One copy of *The Change'll Do You Good* costs $14.95 plus $3.95 for shipping and handling.

Number of books requested: _____

Total Enclosed: _____

Mailing Address:

Name: _____

Address (include zip code): _____

_____

_____

Questions? Call DCS Publishing at:
312-719-9400

Thank you